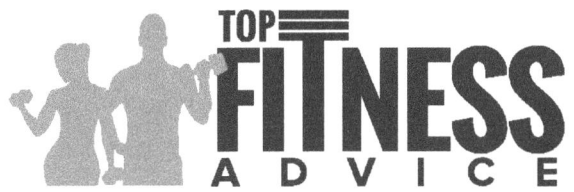

SCREW THE GYM!

The Guide to Losing Weight At Home – NO Gym, NO Expensive Equipment, NO Excuses

Amy Jenkins

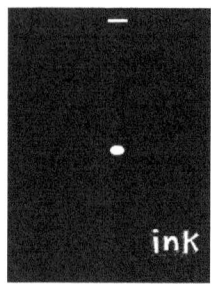

First published in 2017 by Venture Ink Publishing

Copyright © Top Fitness Advice 2019

All rights reserved.

No part of this book may be reproduced in any form without permission in writing from the author. No part of this publication may be reproduced or transmitted in any form or by any means, mechanic, electronic, photocopying, recording, by any storage or retrieval system, or transmitted by email without the permission in writing from the author and publisher.

Requests to the publisher for permission should be addressed to publishing@ventureink.co

For more information about the contents of this book or questions to the author, please contact Amy Jenkins at amy@topfitnessadvice.com

Disclaimer

This book provides wellness management information in an informative and educational manner only, with information that is general in nature and that is not specific to you, the reader. The contents of this book are intended to assist you and other readers in your personal wellness efforts. Consult your physician regarding the applicability of any information provided in this book to you.

Nothing in this book should be construed as personal advice or diagnosis, and must not be used in this manner. The information provided about conditions is general in nature. This information does not cover all possible uses, actions, precautions, side-effects, or interactions of medicines, or medical procedures. The information in this book should not be considered as complete and does not cover all diseases, ailments, physical conditions, or their treatment.

You should consult with your physician before beginning any exercise, weight loss, or health care program. This book should not be used in place of a call or visit to a competent health-care professional. You should consult a health care professional before adopting any of the suggestions in this book or before drawing inferences from it.

Any decision regarding treatment and medication for your condition should be made with the advice and consultation of a qualified health care professional. If you have, or suspect you have, a health-care problem, then you should immediately contact a qualified health care professional for treatment.

No Warranties: The author and publisher don't guarantee or warrant the quality, accuracy, completeness, timeliness, appropriateness or suitability of the information in this book, or of any product or services referenced in this book.

The information in this book is provided on an "as is" basis and the author and publisher make no representations or warranties of any kind with respect to this information. This book may contain inaccuracies, typographical errors, or other errors.

Liability Disclaimer: The publisher, author, and other parties involved in the creation, production, provision of information, or delivery of this book specifically disclaim any responsibility, and shall not be held liable for any damages, claims, injuries, losses, liabilities, costs, or obligations including any direct, indirect, special, incidental, or consequences damages (collectively known as "Damages") whatsoever and howsoever caused, arising out of, or in connection with the use or misuse of the site and the information contained within it, whether such Damages arise in contract, tort, negligence, equity, statute law, or by way of other legal theory.

Table of Contents

Disclaimer — 3

Who is this book for? — 7

What will this book teach you? — 9

Introduction: Why Home Workouts Often Fail, and How to Ensure Your Routine is Always Successful! — 11

Chapter 1: Working Out at Home by Following a Routine — 21

Chapter 2: Pilates and Yoga at Home — 31

Chapter 3: Your Home As Gym Equipment — 39

Chapter 4: Home Chores Are A Workout! — 45

Chapter 5: Inexpensive Equipment to Buy and Use at Home — 51

Chapter 6: Sports, Games, and Other Physical Activity to Try from Home — 57

Conclusion — 65

Final Words — 69

Would you prefer to listen to my book, rather than read it?

Download the audiobook version for free!

If you go to the special link below and sign up to Audible as a new customer, you can get the audiobook version of my book completely free.

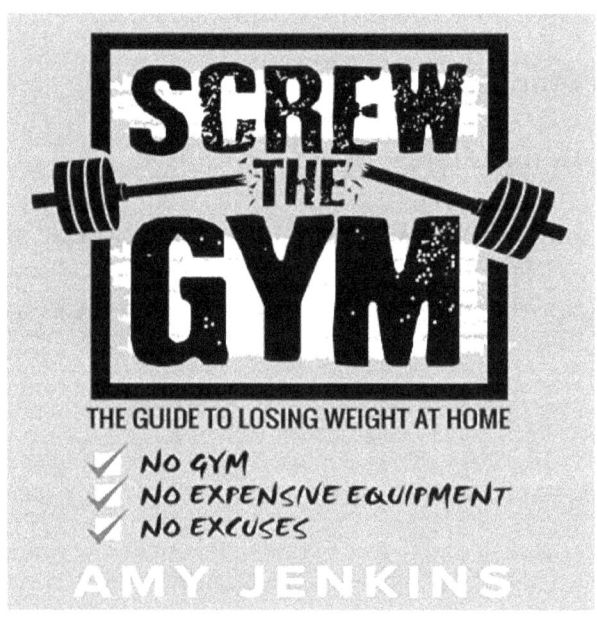

Go here to get your audiobook version for free:

TopFitnessAdvice.com/go/ScrewGym

Who is this book for?

Are you tired of paying for expensive gym memberships with monthly dues that just go up and up every single year, and of visiting the gym only to find that you spend more time waiting in line for a piece of equipment than actually using it?

Do you find it embarrassing to work out in front of others, or get distracted by other gym-goers who want to chat, flirt, or give you unnecessary tips and pointers on your routine?

Do you hate trying to work out in a crowded class, or too often, find that a class has been cancelled or is full so you can't even get in?

Do you avoid going to the gym when it's too cold or too snowy, or when there's too much traffic, or when it's already too late at night by the time you're ready to head out the door?

Do you hate needing to look for a sitter for your children, or spending more time driving back and forth to the gym than you do actually being in the gym?

If so, then this book is for you! We're going to show you how you can get a tough, effective workout right from the privacy and convenience of your own home, with simple equipment you can afford and then store away easily, or without any actual exercise equipment at all.

Forget the expensive membership, heavy traffic, and long lines for equipment at your gym; if you're ready to get started with working out, losing weight, and toning up without ever leaving your home, we're ready to help!

What will this book teach you?

Have you always wanted to ditch those expensive gym memberships and work out from the privacy of your own home, at your own convenience and without long lines, but were worried about how to get an effective workout that really burns calories and builds muscle?

Have you tried to work out at home before, but found that your routine wasn't giving you any results, or didn't know what to do with that expensive and bulky gym equipment after your workout was over?

If so, then you've come to the right place! In this book, we'll teach you, not just how to work out at home, but how to ensure your routine is effective and challenging and really burns serious calories.

We'll also teach you how to working out at home can build real muscle and trim and tone your figure.

You'll also learn the best equipment to use that isn't expensive, that won't take up much room, and which can fit into any home and any routine.

We'll also teach you why so many home workout routines fail, and how to avoid some common mistakes yourself when working out at home, so your routine is always effective and you'll lose weight and then be able to keep it off for good.

If you're ready to learn how you can ditch the gym while still being challenged, while also burning calories and building muscles, let's get started!

Introduction

Why Home Workouts Often Fail, and How to Ensure Your Routine is Always Successful!

If you've tried working out from home before but have had limited or no results at all, or have found that you've even gained weight after giving up your gym membership, there may be a few reasons for this.

It's good to start out this book by examining those reason, as you need to ensure you correct any mistakes you might be making when you ditch the gym and work out from home, or else you'll never get the results you want!

Check out some common reasons for failing to reach your weight loss and fitness goals when you ditch the gym and start exercising at home, and be honest with yourself if any of these apply to you.

Slowing Down

One of the most common reasons that you don't get results when you work out from home is that you soon slow down in your routine.

Consider how this might work when you ditch the gym and follow a routine at home. You might ride an exercise bike when watching your favorite TV program, but soon your pedaling becomes slow and dull as you're not really paying attention to the effort you're exerting, and are distracted by the program. In turn, you're not working your heart and lungs, so you're not really burning calories.

As another example, you might go for a walk after dinner, and this can certainly be a better choice than just plunking down on the sofa for some TV.

However, you may find that soon your brisk walk that once covered several miles becomes a slow walk around the block just once or twice. Again, you're not challenging your heart and lungs, so your results slow down or come to a complete standstill.

Not Challenging the Muscles

Another problem with working out at home is that you soon stop challenging the muscles.

This often happens when a person follows the same routine over and over, so that the muscles they're using get developed and toned and then they're no longer challenged.

When this happens, you aren't burning calories efficiently and aren't going to tone any new muscles, so you see no new results from your workout.

One common reason for this is that you may be relying on the same piece of equipment and may never change up your routine; you may walk on the treadmill or ride that exercise bike every night, and do nothing else to work out.

You may also go at the same pace every time you work out, so your muscles aren't being trained very hard.

Another reason for this happening is that you just aren't exerting yourself and putting in any extra effort during a workout.

Remember that you burn calories when you put in effort for any routine; this can mean running on a treadmill or scrubbing the floors at home, not working at a leisurely pace.

It's not always **what** you're doing that burns calories, but **how much effort** and energy you're putting into that activity. When you're at home, however, it becomes all too easy to start getting downright lazy with your workout, and pretty soon you're seeing few if any results.

Getting Distracted

At the gym, there is usually nothing to do but work out and exercise, and especially if you sign up for a particular class.

However, at home, it's too easy to start thinking about laundry and the dishes that need to be done, or to take a phone call or check your email.

In turn, your workout routine becomes somewhat shortened, or you decide that you'll skip it "one more time," thinking you'll catch up the next day, but soon that one day leads to another missed workout, and another, and so on.

Avoiding These Mistakes!

If these are the most common mistakes made when you ditch the gym and work out from home, how do you avoid them?

Consider a few simple tips to ensure your home workout routine is always effective.

- Keep it upbeat and challenging. No matter what you do for a cardio workout routine, you want to ensure you're always moving fast and working your heart and lungs.

    This is not the time for a leisurely walk around the block or a slow-paced peddle on the bike! Turn off the TV and put down the book if necessary, so you can concentrate on your pace and if you're always pushing yourself.

- Use different equipment and different routines every day. If there is one advantage to working out at a gym, it's that it offers different machines and equipment for working out, so you're always challenging your muscles as you switch up machines, weights, and other equipment.

    When you work out at home, compensate for this by doing something different every day. If you walk on Monday, use the bike on Tuesday and then stair steppers on Wednesday.

    If you don't follow the same routine twice in a row, you're less likely to stop challenging your muscles and will always be pushing yourself and building that muscle tone.

- Use music. Gyms often have fast-paced music pumping through loudspeakers for a reason; it gets your heart rate up and gets you moving so you're less likely to slow down and start getting lazy.

  Use your MP3 player, stereo, computer, or whatever else you need to keep the music pumping while you work out at home.

- Make it downright difficult. When working out at home, think of how to make things downright difficult. If jumping rope makes you short of breath and sweaty, of course you want to be safe, but this is also a good sign that the workout is difficult.

  When scrubbing floors, get down on your knees rather than trying to just bend down. Don't rush up and down stairs but definitely take them two at a time, for an added challenge.

  If something seems difficult and challenging, as long as it's safe for you, this is a good sign for what you should be doing to work out at home.

- Block out time. Treat your home workout as you would an appointment; block out an hour and be determined to do nothing else and think of nothing else but your exercising for that hour.

This includes no checking of the emails or Facebook, or doing "just one simple chore" that could easily lead to a full day of distraction so that you never get back to your routine.

The Importance of Interval Training

Interval training refers to mixing up the pace of your routine and what you're doing during your routine, so that muscles are always "surprised" and, in turn, always challenged. Interval training can be used for any workout routine you choose, even walking or biking.

Consider how interval training works. Start with a scale of 1 to 10 for the amount of exertion you need for any exercise.

For example, when walking, a slow and leisurely walk will be a 1, a brisker pace might be a 3 or 4, jogging might be a 5 or 6, sprints are an 8, and a full-out run is a 10.

Now that you have this scale in mind, you would use interval training when walking by mixing up your pace.

You might walk at a 1 or 2 level to start out, then do a sprint at an 8 level for 30 seconds, then drop down to a brisk pace at a 3 or 4 for several minutes, then do a full-out run at a 10 level for just a few seconds, then jog at a 5 pace for several minutes, and so on.

The key to using interval training successfully is to always incorporate those higher levels or your more challenging pace every few minutes, and not use a slower pace for more than a few minutes either.

This pushes your heart and lungs and keeps your muscles from resting while not allowing yourself to become overexerted.

You also don't want to repeat the same cycle over and over, but mix it up, just as you do your overall routine.

For example, you don't want to simply walk at a brisk 3 or 4 pace for five minutes and then sprint at an 8 pace for 30 seconds, then drop back down to your brisk pace and repeat this again and again.

Instead, go up and down with your pacing, adding in those most challenging speeds as much as possible, but at different intervals and with different intervals following each other. This will ensure you're getting the best workout possible.

Remember, too, that you can use interval training for virtually any routine. If you're biking, increase your pedal speed to go as fast as you can and as fast as is safe, for several minutes during your ride.

Do the same with an aerobics routine you follow at home; ensure you're pushing yourself as fast and as hard as you can with the moves several times during the routine, and you'll have the most success.

Discover Scientifically-Proven "Shortcuts" & "Hacks" to Lose Weight FASTER (With Very Little Effort)

For this month only, you can get Linda Westwood's best-selling & most popular book absolutely free – *Weight Loss Secrets You NEED to Know*.

Get Your FREE Copy Here:
TopFitnessAdvice.com/Extras

Discover scientifically-proven tips to help you lose weight faster and easier than ever before. With this book, readers were able to improve their weight loss results and fitness levels. So, it's highly recommended that you get this book, especially while it's free!

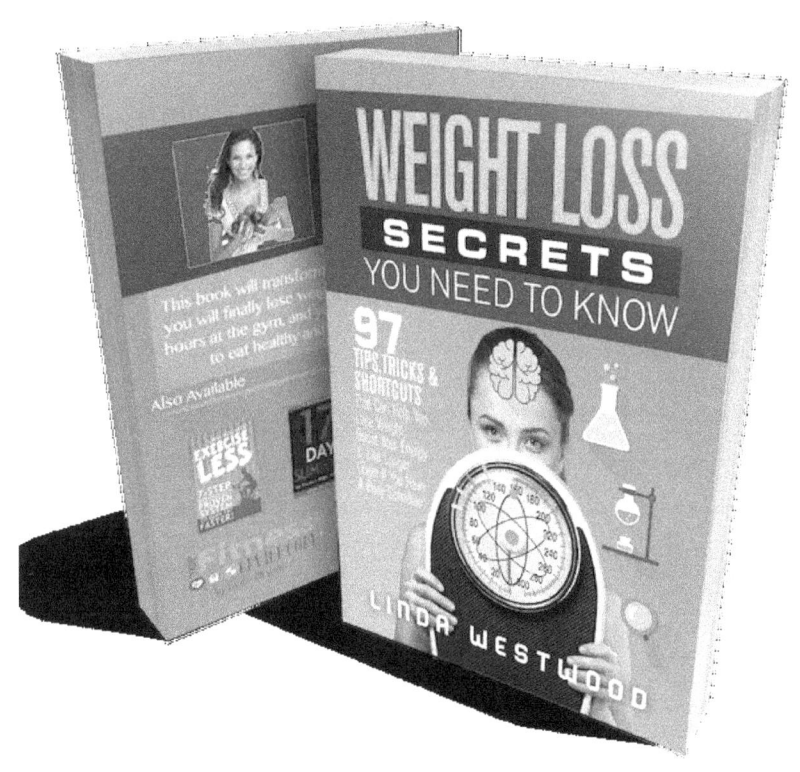

Get Your FREE Copy Here:

TopFitnessAdvice.com/Extras

Chapter 1

Working Out at Home by Following a Routine

A good way to work out at home without having to visit the gym is to create exercise routines that don't require any fancy equipment, including exercise bikes, a treadmill, an elliptical trainer, and the like.

You might dismiss such routines, but keep in mind that members of the military and many professional athletes get a very challenging workout routine without ever using one piece of equipment.

Consider first some classic moves you might try when working out at home.

Classic Moves

First note a few common and classic moves you can do to work out, with or without a set routine, and how to improve them and make them more challenging.

- Jumping jacks. This classic is very good because it burns calories when you jump and also stretches your entire body every time you lift your hands over your head and stretch your legs.

    The most challenging way to perform jumping jacks is to do them quickly, so that you don't even have time to really land and set your feet on the ground between jumps.

- Marching in place. While walking is good, marching is a faster pace that challenges your heart and lungs. Picking up your knees so that your feet are really lifted off the ground makes your body work harder, and also stretches all the muscles in your legs.

- Sprints. Sprints are good for working the heart and lungs, as your body responds to this quick and sudden pace by increasing your heart rate very quickly.

  Sprints are also usually easier to do than running for long distances, while you still burn calories with those short sprints.

- Side stretch. A side stretch is when you stand with your feet shoulder-width apart, arms up by your shoulders. Lean to the left, picking up your right toes as you move your right leg out slightly, reaching your right arm up, to the left, and across your head.

  Return to your starting position and then repeat for the other side, leaning to the right, standing on your left toes as you move your left leg out to the side slightly, reaching your left arm up and to the right, across your head.

  Do these as quickly as possible, not allowing for a rest between each one. These stretches keep you moving and also stretch your sides and legs.

- Pushups. Another classic, these build strong muscles in the arms, back, and shoulders. If you can't do a traditional pushup quite yet, keep your knees on the ground rather than balancing on your toes and hands. This will disperse some of your body weight as you build up the strength in your arms.

- Arm curls. You need free weights to make this move effective, which we'll talk about in the next section. However, arm curls can tone and trim the biceps and all muscles of the upper arms and shoulders, and they're very easy to do.

- Bicep extends. To perform a biceps extend, use a free weight and stand with your right arm extended above you, then bend at the elbow so that your upper arm goes behind you, your lower arm still pointing straight up. Your elbow should be outside the corner of your eye.

  Straighten your lower arm, lifting it into the air, and then lower it back again, and repeat. This move works your entire set of triceps and all muscles in that upper part of your arm.

- Presses. To work the shoulders and upper arms, hold your free weights in your arms with your hands just above your shoulders, about at the corners of your eyes, palms facing outward, keeping your elbows down rather than pointing them in front of you. Raise your hands straight in the air, just as when pushing a bar of weights above you.

- Handstands. A handstand also builds strong muscles in the arms and back, and helps with your posture and balance. You can lean against a wall or have a friend help you get into position and stay balanced on your hands when you're first starting out with a handstand, until you can support yourself fully on your arms alone.

- Lunges. To perform a lunge, stand with your feet shoulder width apart, hands on your hips. Step forward with your right foot and then bend at the knees so that your midsection is being pulled straight down; don't bend forward, putting weight on your right knee, but keep the right leg in a ninety-degree angle.

  Straighten and return to your starting position, then repeat with the other side. This tones and strengthens the legs and backside.

- Squats. Squats build and tone the muscles of the backside and inner thighs.

  To perform a squat, stand with your feet shoulder width apart and lean back slightly, so your weight is on your heels. Bend at the knees so you squat down, still leaning back so your weight isn't supported by your knees.

  Tense the muscles in your inner thighs and buttocks as you push yourself back up to your start position. You can mix up the muscles you work by moving your feet to a wider stance; a sumo squat is when your legs are very far apart, like the stance a sumo wrestler takes.

Mixing up your stance will mean a more thorough workout and more effective squat.

To use these moves for a home workout, create a challenging routine that mixes them up and gives you some variety.

Start with a light jog in place to get warmed up, then do 2 minutes of side lunges, 2 minutes of jumping jacks, 10 pushups, then 10 squats and 10 lunges, as an example, rather than doing just jumping jacks alone.

Vary this routine every day and according to your own fitness levels. You might walk in place for 2 minutes to warm up, then do 10 deep lunges to work the leg muscles, followed by the maximum number of pushups you can manage. Go back to the legs by performing 10 squats.

If you're able to, perform a handstand and hold your weight for as long as possible, then keep up your heart rate by marching in place for 3 minutes. Keep mixing up these moves for a great overall workout.

Following A Routine

If creating a routine with classic moves is a bit overwhelming for you, consider investing in good routines you can follow. There are many DVDs you can purchase with aerobic routines; this includes basic aerobics, military style calisthenics, and everything in between.

If you have cable TV, check out your "on demand" section for aerobic or exercise routines, or you might find daily exercise programs on a sports channel that you can follow at a certain time every day.

There are also routines you can follow from YouTube or other online programs and websites; set up your computer or tablet where you can easily see it and just follow along. You might also be able to purchase a cord that allows your computer to be plugged into your TV, so the TV becomes a computer screen; this can make it easier to see the routine.

As with DVDs, be sure you mix these up and don't follow the same program every day, and you'll be getting a challenging and effective workout that really delivers results.

There are some benefits to following an actual routine with an instructor when you work out at home:

- The routines go for a set time. As said, one challenge many people face when they work out at home is sticking with the routine long enough for it to be effective.

  If you follow a routine online or with a DVD, you know you'll be getting in your full half hour or hour or whatever else you choose, and won't be so tempted to quit early.

- They're safe. Trying to work out at home, on your own, can mean pulling muscles that haven't been properly warmed up or stretched, not cooling down after a workout so the muscles can relax and repair themselves, or performing certain exercises like squats and lunges incorrectly.

Following a routine with a professional instructor will mean being safe while working out at home and reducing your risk of injury.

- They're challenging. As said, it can be a problem with keeping your workout challenging and keeping up with your exertion when you exercise at home. However, if you keep your eyes on the instructor, you can keep pace with him or her and be sure to add that extra effort and energy when needed.

- You're not alone. Working out with a partner can be a great way to stay motivated and keep your routine fun, but you may not always be able to have someone over to play basketball or go with you when you jog.

  Workout routines from a DVD or from an online source usually means more than just the instructor; typically, there is an entire class of persons who are following the routine as well, so you don't feel like you're the only one working out. This can make it more enjoyable and also help you keep up the pace of the routine.

- You can mix it up. As said, invest in a few different DVDs of different types of routines, or find different routines online and follow a different one every day.

  You then won't need to worry about getting too settled in your routine and will know that you're really challenging your muscles by working on something different every day.

Fun Ways to Work Out At Home

If you hate the idea of following a workout routine at home because it starts to get boring, consider a few ways to get your exercise without leaving the house, and without ever getting bored:

- Dance. You don't need expensive dance lessons to dance at home; you can often find lessons online that are easy to follow from home, and you can dance on your own if you don't have a partner.

  Try country line dancing, ballroom dancing, or older classics like the jitterbug to get you moving and get your heart racing! Dance can also be incorporated with aerobic moves for a great workout that is fun and effective.

- Playing with the kids. When was the last time you played "follow the leader" around the house with the kids, or gave them a piggyback ride, or had a game of indoor or outdoor tag? These games can keep you moving and keep you active, indoors or out.

- Outdoor games. Do you have a basketball net over the garage or in the driveway, or a ping-pong table in the garage, or badminton net in the backyard? What about a trampoline?

  These things shouldn't be just for the kids, but take full advantage of them yourself and you might be surprised at how easily you can get your heart going and burn calories while still having fun. We'll talk even more about these choices in another section.

Chapter 2

Pilates and Yoga at Home

Pilates At Home

One of the best routines you can follow at home is Pilates, so it deserves its own section and mention. Pilates is a series of movements that use the body's own weight as resistance, in order to build strong and lean muscles. You can perform a Pilates routine at home with nothing more than an exercise mat, and get a trim and toned figure in no time.

Let's cover some basic Pilates moves so you can follow them at home, and create a simple routine for strong muscles without investing in any weights.

- The swim. To perform this move, lie down on your stomach, arms extended in front of you, legs extended and toes pointed toward the wall.

  Gently kick your legs up and down, keeping them straight and not bending the knees, while moving your arms up and down, as if lightly slapping water under you. This works the buttocks and lower back as they work hard to support you and create those movements.

- The roll. Sit up on your mat and pull your knees to your chest. Wrap your arms around your bent legs and then gently pick your feet up off the ground. Your stomach muscles will immediately tense and flex to keep you balanced. You can hold this pose or add more of a challenge by gently rolling in a small circle.

- Figure 8. Lie down on your back and extend your legs straight up in the air, pointed at the ceiling, feet together; your back and legs should form a 90-degree angle. Gently move your legs, while keeping the feet together, in a figure 8.

  Don't allow your legs to move any wider than your own hips; keep the figure 8 nice and compact. Reverse the direction of the figure 8 to work all the muscles in your back and abdominal area.

- The hundred. This classic Pilates moves really works the belly. Lie on your back, knees bent, feet flat on the ground. Your arms should be by your side but pointing down, toward your feet, not out to the sides. Gently curve your head and neck off the ground while keeping the back of your shoulders on the floor.

  Lift your arms just a few inches off the ground and gently slap them up and down, not touching the floor but just making a slight movement, and count each slap as you go. Try to reach 100 slaps as you keep your stomach muscles tense, holding your head and neck off the ground.

- Bridge. This movement strengthens your lower back and tightens and tones the buttocks and backs of your legs. Lie on your back, knees bent, feet flat on the floor, legs slightly apart. Lift your buttocks and back off the floor so that your body, from your knees to your shoulders, is in one straight line.

Tighten your buttocks as you hold this position for 10 seconds; lower to the ground and rest, then repeat. Don't bounce in and out of this position but move into it smoothly and hold it, keeping the buttocks tense as you do.

- Kneeling side kick. To firm the buttocks and all of the legs, get down on your hands and knees, legs shoulder-width apart. Lift your right leg outward, keeping the knee bent so your knee is now pointed at the wall to your right.

  Gently kick out, or straighten your leg so that your foot points to the right side of you. Bend the knee or pull your lower leg back and return to your starting position, knee on the floor, and repeat. Perform an equal number of reps for each leg.

- Rainbow. While on your hands and knees, extend your right leg behind you and to the right side just slightly, pointing the toes behind you. Gently pick up the leg and move it in an arc behind and across your body, so that it slightly crosses the left leg.

  Don't touch the floor as you continue to move your leg back and forth in this arc, keeping it just a few inches higher than your body. You should feel the buttocks and thighs tense as you perform this movement. Repeat for an equal number of reps for each leg.

Yoga At Home

Yoga is not just some new age fad and it's not about chanting or just getting into odd and difficult positions. True yoga is about concentrating on your movements and poses while stretching all your body's muscles and breathing deeply.

Stretching is good and needed for any exercise routine, as this allows your muscles to take in more blood and oxygen so they can become stronger. Stretching also means you're less likely to pull a muscle or suffer another injury when working out.

Yoga also keeps you flexible so that you can more readily perform certain movements such as stretching and bending, which are needed for a good workout.

Yoga can also improve your posture, which will reduce your risk of injuring your back when you work out.

Consider a few simple yoga moves you might try at home:

- Downward dog. This is a classic yoga move that really stretches the legs and back. Stand with your feet at the corners of your yoga mat and lean forward, gently walking your hands to the opposite corners of the mat.

  Your body should be bent at the hips in a 45-degree angle, so your body and the mat form a triangle. Keep your feet as flat as possible on the mat but relax your back, using your arms and legs to hold your weight.

As you perform this move more often, you'll strengthen and lengthen those leg muscles so you can keep your feet flatter each time, stretching your legs more deeply.

- Seated twist. Sit on your yoga mat, legs bent at the knees, feet flat on the ground. Bend your left leg at the hip, lowering the knee to the ground, keeping your left foot in place under your right leg, as if you were going to sit cross-legged, but keeping your right leg in its position.

  Gently twist at the waist to your right, reaching past your right leg with both arms, touching your right hip with both hands, keeping your left leg lowered and touching the ground.

  You'll feel your right side and back twist gently. Don't bounce or twist back and forth, but simply hold this pose, and then reverse your position and twist with the other side.

- Front stretch. Sit on your yoga mat, legs in front of you and spread so that your feet are actually outside the mat. Very gently lean forward, stretching your arms out in front of you, between your legs, palms on the ground.

  Continue to gently push your arms as far as you can reach, sliding your hands in front of you, to stretch the inside of your legs and your back.

- Cobra. The cobra pose helps to put your spine back in alignment, alleviating pain in the back that you might get with poor posture. Lie on your yoga mat, face down, legs out behind you and only slightly apart, arms at your sides as if you're going to do a pushup. Gently roll up your upper body, starting with your head, then neck, then shoulders, then your hip bones.

Use your arms and hands to keep you in position but remember to roll; you're stretching your upper body backwards, not pushing it off the mat.

Your body should be in a curve off the mat, your legs still on the ground. To release this position, roll back down, starting with the upper body, then your neck, then your head.

- Child's pose. This pose stretches all your leg muscles and the back. Start on your hands and knees and then bend your knees, moving your upper body back while keeping your hands in the same spot.

  Fold your body so that your buttocks on your heels, while your back, arms, and upper body are stretched out in front of you.

- Tree pose. Tree pose is basically standing on one foot, which sounds very simple, but you may be surprised at how challenging this is to do while keeping yourself balanced and upright!

  Stand with your feet about shoulder width apart and pick one foot off the ground. If you cannot bend the leg enough to rest your foot on the inside of the opposite thigh, avoid tucking that foot against the opposite knee, as this puts pressure on the joint.

Instead, tuck it behind the opposite leg. You may need to keep your hands on your hips or in front of you, palms together, until you can master this move, but for the most stretch, lift your arms straight up in the air, keeping your face forward.

For an added stretch, put your arms behind your back and clasp your hands, then stretch your arms downward and out behind you.

To ensure that your yoga routine is safe as well as successful, note a few simple but important tips.

- Always roll, never bend, and move gently. Yoga is not about burning calories through exertion but involves gently stretching of the body.

   For all your moves, and especially when switching between moves, gently roll your body into position rather than bending the back or neck.

   Bending can pull muscles whereas rolling means a gentle stretch. Be sure you move slowly and gently when you do change positions so you don't put pressure on the joints.

- Hold poses, don't bounce or repeat them quickly. Stretching your muscles is best done when you get into a stretching pose and then hold it, rather than bouncing back and forth.

This bouncing can injure muscles and also put pressure on the joints. Again, yoga is not to be confused with aerobics, but is just for a stretch, not a workout.

- Relax your muscles. While Pilates and other routines involve tensing muscles to make them stronger, you need to concentrate on relaxing muscles during yoga.

  This will keep them open to the added blood and oxygen that flow through them when you stretch them, and ensure you're not putting pressure on the muscles that could cause injury.

- Hold poses as is comfortable. Stretching deeply will help bring in more blood and oxygen, as will holding poses for several minutes, but try yoga at your own pace and as is safe for you.

  For instance, if you can't bend your leg when you try tree pose to tuck it behind the opposite leg, tuck that foot behind the opposite ankle and stand in that pose just as long as possible; do the same for all your other stretches.

  Don't get discouraged, as you'll soon be able to increase your stretching and time you hold your pose if you keep up with your yoga routine.

I hope that you are enjoying this book so far, and if you could spare 30 seconds, I would greatly appreciate you leaving a review on Amazon.com.

Chapter 3

Your Home As Gym Equipment

What does it mean that your home is gym equipment? Quite simply, there are many items around your home that you can use as gym equipment in order to get an effective and challenging workout, without spending a dime on gym membership or for investing in new equipment!

Consider a few suggestions for how you can use everyday items in place of gym equipment; of course, always be mindful of safety and wear "grippy" shoes that give you good traction, and ensure all items you use are in good repair and free of obstacles or anything that might get in the way of your workout or that would cause injury.

Stairs

Using a stair machine at the gym is a great way to work out all the muscles in the legs while improving your posture and balance, and challenging your heart and lungs. If you have a set of stairs at home, either indoors or out, then you've got a stair machine you can use!

Be very careful about using actual stairs as no workout is worth a fall, and tumbling down even a few steps can mean twisting an ankle or suffering an even worse injury. Make sure stairs are clear of all debris and that any carpet on the stairs is not loose.

Don't pull yourself up by the handrail as this takes some of the effort away, but don't hesitate to lightly grip or touch the rail to keep yourself balanced and safe. You also want to ensure you push yourself up with your leg muscles, not your knees, to avoid injury and fatigue on that joint.

The stairs are also not the place to get "fancy" by high-stepping, marching, or taking too many steps at a time, and especially if you're trying to increase your speed. However, using a brisker pace when going up and down stairs can really work the heart and lungs and burn lots of calories.

You can also use the stairs as a stepper, not running up and down the staircase but just stepping up onto the second or third stair and then lowering yourself back down, and then switching legs.

This movement works the muscles of the legs and buttocks. Be sure you lean back just slightly when you do this, putting your weight on your heels and not your knees, while not leaning so far back that you might actually fall off the step!

Sprints

Sprints are very good for burning calories as we've already mentioned, and the good news is that you don't need a lot of room to perform effective sprints!

If you have a long hallway, basement, great room, or even some space outdoors, you can perform short sprints from one side to another and increase your heart rate to burn maximum calories.

As with stairs, make sure you have a clear path to run sprints and there is no loose carpeting or other obstacles. Start slowly so you get a feel for the area in which you'll be sprinting and then work up to faster speeds; try to avoid stopping before you turn and sprint the other way, to keep your heart rate elevated and burn maximum calories!

Weights

To build muscle, you need some resistance, and that often means weights. How do you use household objects as weights?

Lifting heavy objects alone isn't always the solution, as some objects might not be balanced in their weight or easy to lift, so that you wind up using your back muscles or being slightly off balance when you lift those items, and this can lead to injury.

Good items to use are those that are easy to hold in your hand but which you can make heavier as needed. As an example, take an old soup can and fill it with wet sand, then cover the top with tin foil and secure the foil with a rubber band around the can. You now have a free weight you can easily hold in one hand!

Similar items include the can you get when you purchase tennis balls; fill this with water, wet sand, kitty litter, gravel, or another item that allows you to control the weight of the can, put the lid back on it, and you have a great free weight.

For something even heavier, save a 2-liter or 1-liter soda bottle after it's empty and fill it with water or wet sand. This fits easily in the palm of your hand and holds more of any type of filler, including water or wet sand, so it can give you a very challenging workout.

To build muscles of the legs and backside, find a heavy book that you can balance on the front of the legs, around your ankles. Lie down on your back, feet together, and put the book on your lower legs, just above your feet.

Lift your feet a few inches in the air; this works your stomach muscles and the weight of the book makes it even more challenging to stay balanced.

You can also use the book in the flat palm of your hand as a free weight, or have a friend put the book on the small of your back when you're ready to do pushups, for added resistance and more of a challenge.

Another idea for a free weight uses a large zipper bag that you can close securely. Fill it with wet sand, wet kitty litter, gravel, or whatever else you can keep inside, and close it up.

You can put this on the small of your back, just like the book, or on your ankles. You can also hold the middle of it like a free weight to do arm curls and other simple movements.

Once again, thank you for reading this book, and I hope you're getting a lot of valuable information. I would greatly appreciate it if you could take 30 seconds to leave me a review for this book on Amazon.com.

Enjoying this book?

Check out our other best sellers!

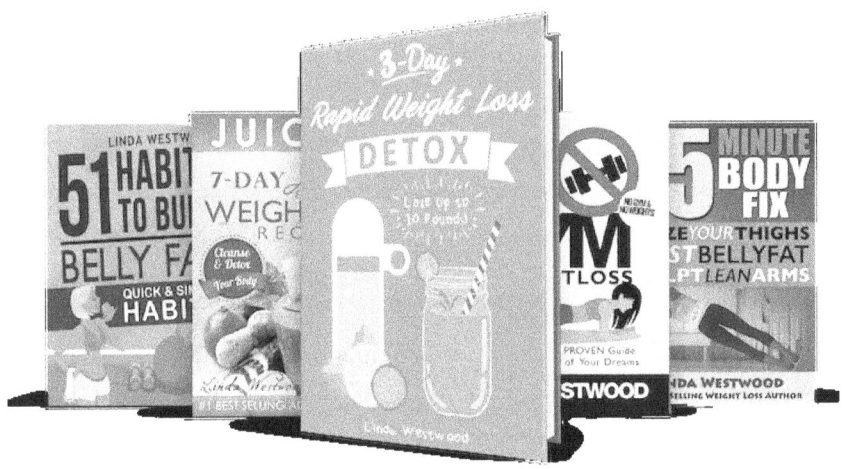

Get your next book on sale here:

TopFitnessAdvice.com/go/books

Chapter 4

Home Chores Are A Workout!

Using your home as a gym doesn't always mean following a standard routine or using gym equipment. If you've ever put in a full day of working around the house and felt tired and sore at the end of that day, then you know that home chores are quite the workout on their own!

Consider a few tips on how to make your everyday chores, and some special chores that you don't normally tackle every day, a full workout that help to burn calories and even build muscle.

Lifting Heavy Weights

Many home chores involve lifting heavy weights that you don't normally lift every day; when you flip mattresses, rearrange furniture, or carry heavy cleaning supplies up and down stairs, you're giving your muscles quite the workout.

You always want to be safe when lifting heavy weights in any circumstance, but lifting or moving these types of items around the house can be a workout that rivals any gym!

Remember that you don't need to wait until you want to rearrange your space to move furniture around the house; three or four times every week, move around the furniture in your living room or dining room, and then put it back again!

Remember that the goal is to work out and get in some resistance training, so don't waste time telling yourself that it's "pointless" to move these items around, but do some carrying of the furniture and other pieces for an hour or so, several times every week.

Vigorous Chores

Vigorous chores can give you a good workout through the day, as you increase your heart rate and really challenge yourself while cleaning or working around the house.

Consider a few examples; scrubbing the bathroom including the shower area and floor, scrubbing the kitchen floor by hand, vacuuming every inch of the carpeting including around the baseboards and up the corners of walls and stairwells, mopping the basement floors, washing windows and walls, or organizing heavy and bulky items in the garage or basement.

You may not look forward to doing these types of chores, but consider how they can be a great workout.

You're stretching every muscle of the body while moving vigorously when you scrub floors and walls, and are giving your muscles a workout as you mop, wash, and scrub, or lift and move around those bulky objects that need some organizing.

As with moving around furniture and other heavy items, don't think about whether or not the bathroom needs to be cleaned or if the walls need washing; schedule a different room you'll tackle every day or every other day, and clean it vigorously from top to bottom, even if it's already clean.

Wash the walls, climb up on a stool to dust light fixtures or ceiling fans, get down on your hands and knees to wash floors, and empty out cupboards to give them a good scrub. If you do this regularly, you'll get a good workout and will also love the look of your spotlessly clean home!

Heavy Chores

Heavy chores are a bit different than vigorous chores, as these require more than just a bit of strength and energy.

Heavy chores might include digging up weeds in a garden or digging a trench or pit for a new landscaping feature, manually sanding down furniture or other items for repainting, refinishing floors, cutting firewood or trimming trees on the property, or cutting the grass with a push mower rather than a power mower.

These heavy chores might not be something you can manage every day, but consider how you can include them in your routine every week or as often as possible.

Start with working outside. You might choose one area of your property that you can dig up and then refill, and then dig up again.

As with other chores, you may not need this digging work done, but remember that you're doing this for a workout, not to dig a pit in your lawn!

Invest in a manual, push lawnmower and use that when it's time to cut the grass, opt for a standard snow shovel versus a snow blower in wintertime, and an old-fashioned rake versus a leaf blower during autumn months.

If your property is looking a little less than presentable, consider how you can combine a good workout with the work needed to be done to get it in great shape!

Buy some manual shears and trim those hedges by hand every week, and a manual edger you can use to go over the borders of your lawn.

Pull weeds, prune trees, and plant new landscaping features. These jobs are all hard work that add up to a very effective workout, and a great looking property is just a bonus!

Exterior cleaning is also a great workout. Get an exterior scrub brush and scrub the deck, the outside of the house and garage, the garage floor, and the driveway. Fire your pool cleaner and clean the pool yourself every week.

In the home, think about big jobs you can tackle that will mean a good workout while also sprucing up the look of the home.

When was the last time you painted the concrete basement floor, sanded and put a coat of sealant over the wood floors, or scrubbed the carpeting by hand?

These heavy chores are about more than just making your home look its best; they'll get you up and moving and work out virtually every muscle of your body!

Tips for Making Chores Work As A Workout

Just doing household chores themselves won't give you a good workout automatically; chances are, you've been doing household chores for years and are still looking to lose some weight and tone your muscles!

To turn your home into a gym and use those chores as an effective workout routine, note a few simple tips to keep in mind:

- Set a timer. Remember that using household chores to get fit is not about working around the house, but is about getting in the exercise you need.

  Set a timer or time for yourself to work around the house and don't stop until that time is up, even if it means vacuuming the same set of stairs one more time or washing the same windows again and again!

- Exert some effort. Normal sweeping and mopping may not burn a lot of calories, but when you increase your pace, use lots of physical exertion when scrubbing, or otherwise exert as much effort as possible, you'll be burning more calories and toning your muscles as well.

- Use music. Don't get distracted by the television, although you can have it on in the background if you're not likely to sit down and start watching.

If that temptation is too much for you, then just use music instead. Keep it upbeat so you keep up your energy levels.

- Turn off the computer. When you're at home, no matter what you're doing, it's often easy to get distracted with Facebook, emails, and everything else online.

   Shut off the computer entirely during your home workout so you're not alerted to new messages or get tempted to spend time online and not with your workout routine.

Others who are considering purchasing this book would love to know what you think. If you could spare a few seconds, they would greatly appreciate reading an honest review from you. Simply view the page on Amazon.com.

Chapter 5

Inexpensive Equipment to Buy and Use at Home

You don't always need actual workout equipment to get in a good, effective routine from home, but sometimes there are small, affordable, and versatile pieces of equipment you might consider, in order to enhance your overall routine.

Consider a few of those here so you can decide if you want to invest in these and make your home workout even better and more effective!

Free Weights

You may not want your home to be cluttered with a complete stack of free weights, but note that you can invest in just one set that is challenging to you, and use only that set for arm curls and presses.

The weight you choose will probably be sufficient for quite some time, so don't assume that you'll always need to keep upgrading to a heavier weight for a good workout routine. Mix up the workouts you follow and how you use the weights, and just one set should be all you need.

Resistance Bands

More compact and easier to store away than free weights, resistance bands can be used to tone arms and legs very easily.

You can simply stretch them apart to work your arms, or tie the ends to your ankles and stretch your legs for a good workout.

Most resistance bands are sold in sets of light to heavy resistance, so you can stock up on a variety and find just the weight and resistance you need for your workout routine.

Steppers

Stepping up onto any surface is a good workout because your legs actually work very hard to push your body weight up; you're actually fighting gravity every time you step up, even a short distance!

It's believed that your legs lift about 3 times your body weight when you step, so stepping up is a great way to tone and firm your leg muscles and burn calories.

While going up and down the steps at home can give you a good workout, this can be very unsafe and, if the only steps you have are outside on your porch, they can be impossible to use during inclement weather. You might also live in a ranch style home with no steps!

Steppers or stepping platforms are a great choice for any home and they come in a wide variety of styles and heights.

Some platforms are wide but not very deep; these are good for aerobic classes, as you can easily alternate your feet when stepping onto a wider platform.

You might also jump up and over the stepper when it's not very deep. These platforms may also come with stackers that you add to each end so you can increase the height of the step itself.

Plyometrics platforms are also a good way to add stepping to your routine. These platforms are typically used for jumping and they may be staggered in height, usually coming in sets of four; the lowest may be 12 inches, then 18 inches, then 24 inches, and then 36 inches off the ground.

While you may not be ready for a full plyometrics routine, investing in the 12-inch or 18-inch platform can mean being able to easily step up without any type of stairs.

Jump Rope

Jumping rope is a very effective workout because, like stepping, you are actually fighting very hard when you lift your entire body off the ground. Your muscles get a good workout and the routine of jumping rope also burns lots of calories.

It's also good to remember that a jump rope takes up virtually no space in your home! You can even use a clothesline when it's not laundry day or any other type of rope that you can safely jump.

Be sure there is nothing around you when you use the jump rope, as it's easy to snag a light fixture or items on a nearby table, but you only need an open space in one room and thick-soled shoes, along with your rope, to get in a great workout.

Exercise Ball

A large exercise ball is great for working the abdominal muscles, as you need to work the abs to keep yourself balanced on the ball.

Doing sit-ups on an exercise ball will also work the back muscles and everything around your core or midsection.

Invest in an exercise ball you can easily deflate and that comes with its own air pump, so you don't face the cost of an electric air pump just to inflate your exercise ball.

Mini Trampoline

You may not have room on your property for a full trampoline, but a mini trampoline can easily be stored under a bed or in a closet when not in use. As with jumping rope, you're giving your body a great workout when you jump up and down on the trampoline.

The trampoline surface itself also helps to absorb some impact, as you're not landing on the hard surface of the ground every time you jump.

This can make a mini trampoline a great choice for those with bad knees or problems with other joints, or who are carrying so much extra body weight that jumping rope could be very dangerous and damaging to those joints.

Ab Roller

An ab roller is a very small and simple piece of equipment; it's typically just two wheels connected by a long handle.

To use it, you get on your knees and grip the roller in your hands in front of you, and then roll while stretching your back, going back and forth.

This works the abdominals and back muscles because they're working very hard to balance you and control your movements as you move back and forth.

Hula Hoop

You may think a hula hoop is just for the kids, but this hoop can build strong abdominal muscles and also be used for the arms and legs.

If you're not very good with a hula hoop, remember to stand up straight and keep your stomach and back muscles tense while you gently gyrate in a small circle; don't try to force the hoop with a wide, swinging motion.

You can also use the hula hoop on your arms and legs; place it over your arm, a safe distance from your face, and give it a twirl to build strong arm muscles.

Lie down on the floor and lift one leg in the air and put the hoop around the lower leg and twirl it, and this will work the thighs, hips, and all the muscles of the leg.

I hope you have learned something from this book so far and would greatly appreciate it if you could leave an honest review on Amazon.com.

Chapter 6

Sports, Games, and Other Physical Activity to Try from Home

Working out in your own home is very good and can be very effective, but you might want to also get outside the house for some fresh air and to ensure your routine doesn't get stale and boring.

Sports and other physical activity are great ways to do this; if you haven't thought about playing any type of sports and don't know where to begin, consider a few suggestions, and then tailor these to your own current fitness levels, schedule, and budget, and of course to whatever else is needed to ensure you stick with your activity and maintain your weight loss goals!

Get A Bike

If you don't own a bike, now's the time to get one; you don't need an expensive mountain bike with lots of gears and other fancy features to get a good workout from a ride.

Buy a used bike you find online to save money, and then set aside a few hours every week to explore the neighborhood, or ride up to a nearby school with a track and ride around the track.

You might also find excuses to ride in order to get more exercise. Put a basket on your bike and you can use it for errands; do you just need a carton of milk from the corner store or to pick up your prescription from the nearby pharmacy? Take your bike rather than the car.

If the kids want to go to a friend's house, have everyone ride their bikes; you can then ride home, then ride back to the friend's house when it's time for the kids to come home.

You'll save money on gas and some wear and tear on your car when you use your bike for these errands rather than always driving, and will also get in a great workout!

Basketball and Badminton

A basketball hoop is typically very easy to install over a garage or other area of the home, and a badminton set doesn't need a lot of room in the yard either.

You don't need to already be in good physical shape to play a few rounds of either game with the kids or your partner, or just have a friend over for a good workout and game between you.

To make these games more successful, treat them like a league. Set a time every week to play, and be sure you play for a certain amount of time or to a certain score so that you don't quit early.

Keep a long-running scorecard so you can be motivated to improve your game with more effort and exertion, and by expending more energy.

This will help burn more calories and make your workout more successful overall.

Mini Baseball

Think you can't play baseball with the kids because your yard is too small? Well, who says you need a regulation field to enjoy a game?

Get some simple markers for the bases; these can be something as simple as folded dish towels, old books you don't mind getting dirty and torn up, or even your pet's plastic food dish!

Set them around your yard in a mini diamond and use a child's plastic bat and ball to ensure no one hits a ball into a neighbor's yard or smashes a window. They're also more affordable than a real baseball and bat!

Put some effort into running around the bases and chasing after the hit balls so you get in an effective workout.

Soccer

As with baseball, you may not have thought about playing soccer in your yard if your space is limited, but again, you don't need a regulation-sized field to just get in some exercise.

You also don't need an actual soccer net, if your yard has a fence or other barricade to keep the ball from going into the street or a neighboring yard.

You can use something very simple as goal markers, even just marking off sections of the yard with tape or putting tape on the fence to denote the goal area.

Play with a friend or the kids and don't worry too much about regulation rules; just have fun and get active in kicking the ball up and down the "field" and trying to steal it from the opponent while scoring points.

Don't forget to share your thoughts on this book by leaving a review on Amazon.com. It takes just a few seconds.com.

Discover Scientifically-Proven "Shortcuts" & "Hacks" to Lose Weight FASTER (With Very Little Effort)

For this month only, you can get Linda Westwood's best-selling & most popular book absolutely free – *Weight Loss Secrets You NEED to Know*.

Get Your FREE Copy Here:
TopFitnessAdvice.com/Extras

Discover scientifically-proven tips to help you lose weight faster and easier than ever before. With this book, readers were able to improve their weight loss results and fitness levels. So, it's highly recommended that you get this book, especially while it's free!

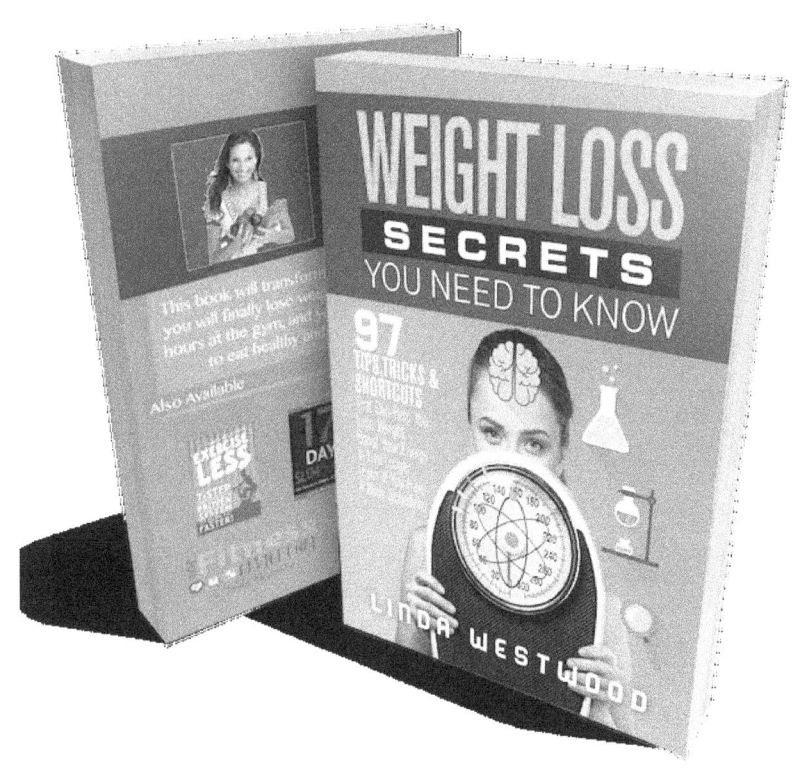

Get Your FREE Copy Here:

TopFitnessAdvice.com/Extras

Conclusion

So, are you ready to ditch the gym and start working out from home? Are you ready to lose weight, build strong muscles, and get yourself heart healthy while also improving your lung health and overall stamina?

Let's review a few key points from this booklet so you can ensure that your home workout routine is the best it can be, and that you can finally see the results you want but without expensive gym memberships and long lines for equipment.

Exert Yourself, Always!

The gym may be a bit stuffy and crowded, but that crowd can help you to stay energized so you're always pushing yourself. Gyms play loud and upbeat music for a reason as well; this is to keep their members in an energized mood so they work hard and see results.

Do the same at home; don't get lazy about your workout but always push yourself so you're burning calories and really working your muscles.

Mix It Up

Doing the same routine over and over again will mean training those muscles so they're not working as hard and, again, you won't be burning calories like you should and won't be building muscle.

Keep track of your routines and what you do every day so you don't repeat the same workout twice in a row, or even fall into a rut of using the same moves and equipment every single day.

It's About The Exercise

If you're going to do some chores around the house to get your exercise, don't think of whether or not the floor is already clean or the walls were scrubbed yesterday; cleaning and fixing up the house isn't really the point.

You can actually just slide heavy furniture around the home and get in a great workout, leaving it right where it started at the end of your workout! Remember that it's about the exercise, not the work to be done, when you work out around the house.

Have Fun

Getting out of the house for a bike ride, to kick a ball around with the kids, or just to go for a light jog for the first time in weeks can be a great way to enjoy your workout. Dancing, using a hula hoop, and other exercises might seem silly but they can also keep your routine fresh and keep you from getting bored and then giving up on your routine altogether.

Keep A Calendar

To make sure that you're not repeating the same workout over and over and are pushing yourself as much as possible, keep a calendar. This should include the routine you follow or the equipment you use, for how long, and how much exertion you used. When you look at this calendar over the course of a week or month, you might see where improvements can or should be made, and your routine will always be fresh and, better yet, effective for weight loss and toning!

Mind Your Diet

While this book is about helping you work out from home so you can ditch the gym and still lose weight and tone muscles, it's worth mentioning that you still need to mind your diet, no matter where and how you exercise.

Exercising, even vigorously, won't allow you to lose weight if you consume more calories than you're burning off. You also need to feed your muscles healthy protein and oils so they can get lean and toned and absorb the vitamins and trace minerals they need.

To help with minding your diet, create a calendar that includes both your everyday eating and exercising. Note your calories, fat, and carbs, and when you eat, so you can see where changes might need to be made.

Cut out the obvious culprits when it comes to losing weight, including sugary sodas and desserts, and snack foods like chips and pretzels that are just empty calories.

If you create a healthy eating plan and make good use of your home for working out and exercising, you're sure to lose the weight, build lean and toned muscles, and keep looking for the rest of your life!

Enjoying this book?

Check out our other best sellers!

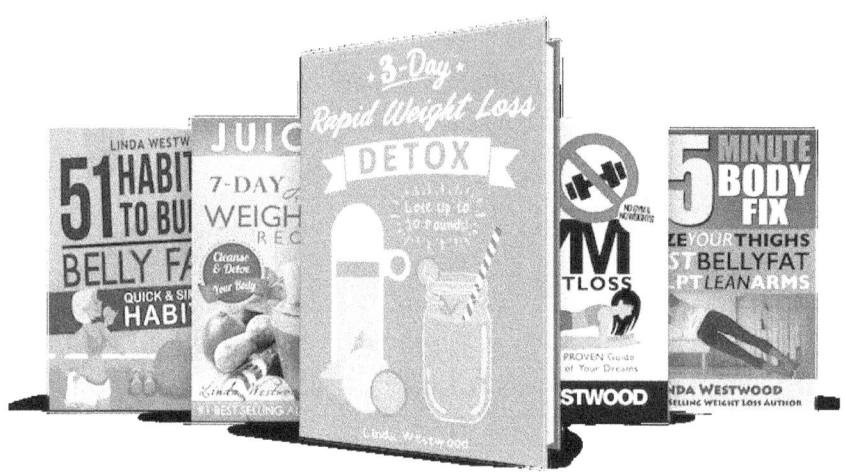

Get your next book on sale here:

TopFitnessAdvice.com/go/books

Final Words

I would like to thank you for purchasing my book and I hope I have been able to help you and educate you on something new.

If you have enjoyed this book and would like to share your positive thoughts, could you please take 30 seconds of your time to go back and give me a review on my Amazon book page.

I greatly appreciate seeing these reviews because it helps me share my hard work.

You can leave me a review on Amazon.com.

Again, thank you and I wish you all the best!

www.ingramcontent.com/pod-product-compliance
Lightning Source LLC
Chambersburg PA
CBHW031209020426
42333CB00013B/858